A BEGINNERS GUIDE TO THE HCG DIET

With Recipes and Meal Plans

By Julia Bond

~~~

The information herein is offered for informational purposes solely, and is universal as so. The presentation of the information is without contract or any type of guarantee assurance.

The trademarks that are used are without any consent, and the publication of the trademark is without permission or backing by the trademark owner. All trademarks and brands within this book are for clarifying purposes only and are the owned by the owners themselves, not affiliated with this document.

TABLE OF CONTENTS

INTRODUCTION

S ince its introduction, the HCG Diet has been receiving widely differing opinions. Some love it while some are adamantly against it.

WHAT EXACTLY IS HCG DIET?

HCG is a hormone naturally produced by the body. It is an important hormone during pregnancy. It also has many other functions outside of pregnancy. Both males and females can benefit from the non-pregnancy-related effects of this hormone.

One of these benefits is weight loss.

How does HCG help with weight loss? Find out in this book.

Here, you will learn:

- What HCG is and how it works in the body

- History of the HCG Diet

- How the diet works

- How the diet plan looks like

- How to properly get started

- How the phases are done

- Tips to food lists

- Recipes

- And so much more

HCG is not a magic fat burning substance. It may be the name of the diet but it is not the single most important element of the diet. Learn more and get a better understanding of this hormone and the diet it is part of.

Read this book today and see how you can lose weight fast safely.

CHAPTER I:
HISTORY OF HCG DIET

HCG was discovered to be effective in inducing weight loss in the 1930s. The exact mechanism is yet to be discovered.

In the 1930s, a study was conducted on obese pubescent boys. Pregnancy hormone was given to these boys. These boys were observed to lose their obesity and developed more muscles. The researchers believed that these observations were caused by isolated HCG.

This result inspired Dr. ATW Simeons to conduct further studies with HCG injections. Obese patients were given a special diet and HCG injections. The results of the study were subsequently published in the infamous manuscript, "Pounds and Inches". This was written in 1971 by Dr. Simeons himself.

After the publication of this manuscript, more studies were conducted on HCG during the 1970s and 1980s. These studies sought either to disprove or prove Dr. Simeons results.

Many studies were unable to reproduce Dr. Simeons. Supporters of the HCG point out a major flaw in these studies. They claim that these studies focused on HCG effect alone, experimented against placebo. HCG proponents claim that it is not HCG alone that produced Dr. Simeons results. It was the special diet that drove the weight loss, augmented by HCG.

CHAPTER 2: GETTING STARTED WITH THE HCG DIET

The HCG Diet can be successful if the protocol is followed. Get accurate baseline data before starting. Baseline data includes weight and similar data. The more comprehensive the baseline data is, the better it will be for evaluating the effectiveness of the protocol. Get measurements such as waist circumference, arms, thighs and hips. Body fat measurements also help.

SCALES AND WEIGHTS

During the program, regular weighing helps. Get a good quality, accurate body weighing scale. You will have to weigh yourself at the same each morning. The best time is right after waking up and getting out of bed. Record each reading. To check progress, weigh yourself upon waking up every day before starting the protocol. This will reflect your baseline weight.

The scale you use before starting the protocol should be the same scale you will use for the duration of the HCG Diet. The scale must be accurate, too. This is important to take note of the fluctuations in weight. This is important so that adjustments in the protocol can be made in time to correct anything that gets in the way of success.

Another important tool is a digital food scale. Digital is more accurate to use. This will be used mostly to weigh the proteins such as chicken, fish and meats. These must be raw when measuring, before the proteins are cooked or prepared into the meal.

PURCHASING HCG

It is best to wait before all the supplies for the HCG Diet are complete before ordering the HCG. Everything must be ready by the time the HCG is ordered and delivered.

Most dieters get their HCG from sellers online. There are many suppliers available, each claiming theirs is legit and highly effective. Research before buying.

Check the reviews on various products and suppliers. This will greatly help you avoid ordering faulty HCG. Worse, some of the products might contain dangerous chemicals. Always be diligent in checking.

Check the website if it is legit. As much as possible, order only from trusted sources. Getting stuff from social network sites might not always be the best practice to get good quality, safe and effective HCG.

OTHER HELPFUL ITEMS

HCG and scales are the most important tools you must have for the diet to be successful. A few other items may also help. Examples are ketone sticks and a grill.

Ketone sticks can help track the body's fat burning rate. These are readily available in many health stores or drugstores.

Grilling is one of the most common cooking techniques you will be using during the diet. HCG diet plan suggests meals that are grilled, broiled or steamed. A grill can help give vegetables added texture and flavor to jazz up meals.

TIPS

Proper preparation is setting up for success. Preparing and starting the diet may be a confusing period. To help, take these tips:

1. Set the goal for losing weight

This is the most important step. Set how much weight you want to lose. It might seem easy to pull off a figure out of thin air. "I'm going to lose 50 pounds in 60 days" is easy to say- but difficult to follow-through.

Weight loss goal must be specific. Set a number. How many pounds exactly?

The goal must be realistic. Sure, there are many incredible stories out there about losing 100 pounds in a short time. It can be possible. However, can your body handle losing that much in such a short time?

Check your health. If you can afford it, have a thorough health check with a physician. Talk about your plan of losing weight to see how much your body can handle. Body transformation can put a strain on your body. Make sure to have a good idea of how much stress your body can effectively handle.

For instance, people with diabetes may not be able to handle severe calorie restrictions. There might be necessary adjustments in food intake as well as dosage of medications. Closer monitoring of sugar levels in the blood may be necessary during the weight loss period.

There are certain health conditions that may not be able to handle drastic weight changes. It is always best to check health status first and gauge if the amount of pounds you want to shed during the program is safe for your condition.

The goal must be attainable. Can you really lose 100 pounds, go from size 6 to size 0 in 60 days? Can you do it? Check your schedule and your own resolve. Write down the reasons why you want to lose that much weight. These will be your motivations to keep you through especially when things start to go rough.

Weight loss goal gives you a tangible finish line. When you record your progress, you know how close you are to where you want to be. This will also help you to keep going and finish the regimen. Your goal will remind you that there is an end to the diet. At the end is something you will really love.

In case you find yourself needing to lose more weight, you can always start another round of HCG safely. You will have to wait a few weeks before starting.

2. Take measurements and picture before starting

These will serve as your baseline data to be used during evaluation. These can help in tracking progress. These can also be motivations of what you do not want to return to.

Suggested measurements to take are not limited to weight. Measure also the thighs, buttocks, waist, around the belly button, chest, neck and arms.

3. Set when to start the diet.

You can start a diet anytime you want. However, to be successful, the start date must be carefully planned. Avoid starting a diet right around the holidays. These will be tempting times to eat and break the diet just when you are starting. Remember, holidays are meant for fun and bonding with loved ones. Food is at the core of these holiday activities. Starting the diet around these times is making the process even more difficult than it should be.

The best time to start the diet is when you have more control over your activities. These should be when your schedule is predictable.

The most recommended periods will be when there aren't scheduled vacations and holidays. Periods when you won't be spending much time outside the home are also great times to start the diet.

Unpredictable schedules can easily derail your carefully created meal plans. An unscheduled dinner meeting or trip out of town can easily put you on the course to eating things not allowed in the diet.

Aim to start the diet when you are pretty sure you can spend the next two months dedicated to transforming your body through the HCG Diet.

4. Choose the type of HCG

People react differently to different forms of HCG. Some achieve success with HCG injections. Some achieve fast results with homeopathic HCG drops while some do well with prescription-grade drops. Choose the right one for you.

How to choose the right HCG for you

Choosing is mainly based on how much weight you need to lose. This is why it is important to prepare well for the diet. The right form will increase the chances for success with the diet. Getting the right form of HCG at the start of the diet is much better at getting results than having to change forms in the middle of the plan.

Get the current weight and compare to the target weight. Compute the difference to get how much weight you need to lose.

High weight loss goals mean needing to lose 25 pounds or more. The right type of HCG is prescription-grade HCG diet drops. The natural design of this HCG form ensures the most efficient fat burning process. The design is meant to target large amounts of stored fats for distribution and burning.

Prescription-grade HCG diet drops also serve as a trigger for suppressing appetite. It is also an energy enabler and a muscle cell protector. These actions make the prescription-grade type as the most effective for those who are starting with HCG drops.

For low weight goals, the target is to lose less than 25 pounds. People who are near their weight loss goals are also considered under this category. The most effective HCG form to use is homeopathic HCG drops. The body can be stimulated to burn off large fat stores. However, if there is a smaller amount of fat left to burn, the body will be reluctant to do so. This is a normal bodily reaction to protect itself from losing too much of its stored energy sources. This is also often triggered when the body loses large amounts of fats over a short period.

Ever noticed people who lost weight and still retain a very noticeable belly bulge? It serves as protection for the internal abdominal organs and as the last resort energy source in case the body experiences extreme starvation over a prolonged period.

To keep the body burning that "last mile" of fat, take homeopathic HCG drops. This formulation includes additional fat-busting boosters. These ingredients signal the body that it is OK to continue burning the fats.

To override this self-preserving instinct, the homeopathic HCG drops will send signals to the body that it is not being starved. Hence, it is OK to let go of these stubborn fats. This type of HCG also gives the body the important nutrition it needs. This serves as sort of a reassurance to the body that it isn't experiencing starvation.

During this phase, the body is not just burning off fats. It is actually undergoing a transformation. The fats burned are from hard-to-reach areas. These are places where the body stores fats fast and reluctant to burn. These fats can be considered as the body's hoard meant to be slowly burned during times of extreme starvation. Example of such places is the belly area.

Another benefit from homeopathic HCG drops is its protective effects on the muscles. Too much fat burned over a short period also triggers the body to start metabolizing the muscles. It starts to breakdown the protein stores in the muscle tissues to provide nutrients and energy. It's another response meant to supply the body with nutrients and energy in times of prolonged starvation. Homeopathic HCG drops protects the muscles from breakdown while boosting the body's energy levels. These help towards body transformation where you have lean muscles, ideal body fat composition and excellent energy levels.

5. Ordering HCG

You do not just order and stack large amounts of HCG. You have to order just enough for a specific phase. This will save you more money and stress from figuring out what to do with all the excess or having several bottles of expired HCG. This will also save you from a bad situation where you need to wait a few days to a week waiting for HCG replenishment. This waiting period of going without HCG can set you back significantly in your HCG diet program.

Uninterrupted HCG use is a key factor in a successful HCG diet program. Order enough HCG for the diet's time-frame.

Ordering in bulk is highly recommended. Spoilage is not going to be an issue. Prescription HCG drops are shipped unmixed. Once opened, these should be refrigerated. Opened, properly refrigerated prescription HCG drops last for 60 days before expiring. This is also the exact time for you to consume it all and complete the HCG regimen.

Homeopathic HCG drops are shipped already mixed. These can be taken as it is. These have a long shelf-life. It can last throughout the entire regimen before expiring.

6. Check the diet plan

HCG comes with a set of diet plan and recommended instructions for use. These come from the supplier. If not, better look for HCG with supplier's diet guidelines.

Review these guidelines. Incorporate these guidelines when you plan your diet regimen. Following the supplier guidelines will increase your chances for success.

7. Evaluate your food supply.

Check all the food you have on hand. Take out everything that looks suspiciously unhealthy. Check the list of approved foods under the HCG Diet plan. Remove everything that isn't on that list.

This is an important step before you start the diet. Remove all temptations now. That box of chocolate chip cookies will be harder to resist the deeper you get into the diet.

Start stocking your pantry and your fridge with the approved foods. Take this opportunity to stock as much as you can. This will save you more trips to the store. This make it easier for you to concentrate on what you should be doing instead of stressing yourself with shopping for the right foods later. You will be less exposed to temptations in the store, too.

8. Start keeping a weight loss journal.

People think that a weight loss journal is just an extraneous activity. Studies prove otherwise. Journals help dieters lose double their weight loss goals compared to those who did not keep a journal.

Keeping a journal is not limited to pen and paper. You can use online journals. There are also downloadable apps meant for keeping journals.

What to put in a journal? Start by writing down foods and the sizes of the portions you consumed throughout the day. Beside these entries, write down how you felt before eating and after eating. This will not only help you keep track of what you eat. This will also help you address emotional eating. This is a growing epidemic that predisposes many of the population to problem like obesity and diabetes.

9. Plan meals.

Start creating a meal plan before you even start the diet. This will help you see that removing a lot of the things you are used to eating is not that bad at all. You still have many options.

10. Plan reward or gorge days.

Incorporate days when you can eat anything you want. Put 2 gorge days on your diet plan. This is a serious thing. Never skip your gorge days as just you must not skip your HCG days.

These gorge days will help ease the challenges you might encounter. Cravings are among the greatest hurdles in the diet. These can be kept under control if you carefully plan your gorge days.

CHAPTER 3:
HOW DOES
THE HCG DIET WORK

HCG is a natural hormone. This human chorionic gonadotropin hormone basically changes how the body loses weight. This is a pro-hormone present in both men and women. Women produce larger amounts of HCG during the pregnancy period. As a pro-hormone, HCG serves as a catalyst hormone stimulating the body to produce other hormones. These other hormones affect metabolism, digestion, muscle tissues, liver functioning and other important bodily processes.

Excess fat storage and obesity are closely linked to hormonal functions and balance of these functions between several different types of hormones. Obesity develops when hormones are not functioning well or when the balance between the hormones is disrupted.

HCG serves as a vehicle to bring balance into the body's delicate hormonal system. Once balance is restored, the body will be able to perform its many functions more efficiently. One of which is efficient metabolism, fat storage and at burning.

FAST FACTS ABOUT HCG

The human chorionic gonadotropin is produced in large amounts by the chorion. This is one of the three layers of the placenta. The placenta is formed within the woman's uterus after an embryo has implanted on the uterine wall. All throughout the pregnancy, HCG serves to control other hormones.

HCG also serves as a precursor molecule to LH and FSH. Leuteinizing hormone and follicle-stimulating hormone control many other hormones, including hormones that regulate metabolism. Higher levels of HCG allow LH and FSH levels to go higher than normal (non-pregnant state). This prevents the stimulation of a negative feedback loop in the hormonal control system. This feedback loop serves to keep hormones from getting too high. During pregnancy, certain hormones need to be higher than normal to support the development of the fetus. HCG allows these hormones to get higher.

This same effect is observed in males and females when HCG levels are high. Certain hormones go higher than the normal range. How high hormones can get elevated depends on the amount of HCG taken.

HCG is approved by the US FDA as a fertility drug. Large doses of about 10,000 IU are given to females to stimulate FSH spikes. This triggers ovulation, which helps those who have ovulatory disorders or help increase chances for getting pregnant.

Males are also given large doses to stimulate dramatic increases in testosterone levels. This results in the direct stimulation of the Leydig cells within the testes. This stimulation helps increase sperm production. In this capacity, HCG is used in males to treat low sperm count.

HCG is also known to cause weight loss. The direct use of HCG as a weight loss agent has yet to receive FDA approval.

How weight loss happens

The body becomes less efficient in using fat for energy if it is out of balance. The imbalances create pauses in the natural bodily processes. These imbalances are usually simply caused by not enough amounts of a nutrient.

For example, when the liver does not receive enough choline, it becomes unable to process fats from food. If there aren't enough of certain hormones, the digestive system will be unable to digest, emulsify and process fats. These can all lead to improper fat metabolism, increased fat storage, poor fat expulsion and difficulty burning fats.

HCG comes in to help.

The HCG diet is not about taking HCG and watching the fat melt away. The diet is all about the food.

HCG is added to change the way the body loses weight. One way is stimulating the glandular follicles. These help in maintaining the muscle tissues.

This is an important step when trying to lose weight. This is especially helpful when losing a large amount of weight.

The body instinctively go into "diet mode" when large amounts of weight are lost rapidly. The result is slower metabolism and increased fat storage. Fats around the belly area become harder to burn. The body even adds more fat in this area.

To keep the body from entering this condition, HCG stimulates the natural metabolic cycle. It maintains muscle mass, which will signal the body that there is no threat of starvation. This reassurance tells the body that it is OK to keep metabolism proceeding at normal pace. HCG also stimulates the normal hormonal cycle, keeping it from changing its course despite the low calorie intake and increased fat burning rate.

On the other hand, most other diets rely mainly on food and calorie restrictions. These will signal the body's preservation mode resulting in slower metabolism. Worse, some of these other diets trigger processes that use muscle tissues as source of energy. This is called starvation mode.

This is also one of the reasons why most other diets fail.

Most people complain they only get to enjoy weight loss for a few weeks then a plateau happens. Worse, they gain back all the weight they lost and then more.

Again, this is a response to the loss of weight and muscle mass. The body slows down metabolic rates and increases fat storage.

CHAPTER 4:
HCG DIET PLAN

Meal plans are usually limited to each meal including a fruit, a piece of bread, a vegetable and 1 portion of lean protein.

You do not eat just about anything. Meals must contain only those in the diet's approved list. It must also be taken in specific amounts.

The HCG Diet is an extreme type of diet. It can result in rapid weight loss of about 1 to 2 pounds in just a day. Another astonishing fact is that you are supposedly not going to feel hungry during the diet.

The diet is composed of 2 major features. It has a super limited calorie restriction to just 500 calories a day. It also has the daily administration of HCG hormone. The hormone is traditionally administered via injections. Today, the hormone is available in serval forms. It is available as oral drops, sprays and pellets.

The HCG Diet is composed of 3 phases. There is the loading phase, the weight loss phase and the maintenance phase.

In the *loading phase*, daily HCG is initiated. The diet is composed of high calorie, high fat foods. This phase lasts for 2 days only. This diet plan is designed to help the body get used to the presence of HCG and its effects.

In the *weight loss phase*, HCG is continued. The diet is limited to 500 calories only per day. This phase is also called the burning phase. The body is stimulated to burn fats. This is through a very low calorie diet or VLCD.

This phase lasts for 3-6 weeks, depending on how much weight needs to be lost. For small weight loss goals, 3 weeks on the weight loss phase should be enough. For those with large weight loss goals, 6 weeks is recommended. Some may have to repeat the cycle a few more times, going through all the 3 phases repeatedly.

During this phase, only 2 meals are taken each day. Usually, this is lunch and dinner only. You may choose what meals to take but it must be the same pair every day for the entire phase. If you started with lunch and dinner only, it must be lunch and dinner for the entire phase. You may also choose breakfast and lunch only or breakfast and dinner only.

In the *maintenance phase*, HCG is discontinued. Food intake is gradually increased. Starch and sugar are avoided. This phase lasts for 3 weeks.

Sometimes, you might achieve your weight loss goals before the minimum 21 days in the burning phase. Complete the 21 days minimum for the burning phase. You may increase your calorie intake a little while completing the minimum period.

If you have been on the burning phase for 42 days maximum and the weight loss goals are not yet achieved, stop and move on to the maintenance phase. Never extend the burning phase beyond 42 days. If there is still some weight to lose, take a break after the maintenance phase then repeat the entire 3 phases of the HCG diet.

Things to consider

This is an extreme diet. Anyone who plans to follow this protocol must consult a doctor first. This is a must for those with existing health concerns.

For women, start the HCG diet immediately after a menstrual period. An alternative starting date will be at least 10 days before the next menstrual period begins. Never start during or before a period.

During the HCG diet, follow these guidelines:

- Take the HCG drops 3 times per day. On the 7th day, do not take any HCG. The next day, take HCG as usual.

- Always weigh yourself every day. The best time to weigh is in the morning. The weight during this time of the day is the most significant as it will reflect a more accurate body weight. The weight typically fluctuates throughout the day. These fluctuations are typically caused by extraneous factors such as water retention. This will not be a reliable gauge of your weight loss progress.

CHAPTER 5:
PREPARING FOR THE DIET

This is the fun part of the diet plan. Preparing for the diet is considered as the diet's Phase 1 or the Loading Phase. This is the part where you can actually enjoy eating because you can eat the foods you love the most.

Eat fatty, calorie-rich foods. Eat to capacity. Eat to your heart's content. BUT.... do not eat until you get sick. Just eat until you are full. Do not stuff yourself to the point of sickness.

Take advantage of the loading phase. This is the only phase when you can overeat. Eat the things you love, even the most fattening ones. Pizza, fatty cuts of meat, pasta, rich desserts- eat up.

Why?

The point of the loading phase is to restore any fat reserves missing in the body at this point. The essential fat reserves are the fats that the body needs for protection and for its many homeostatic functions. You see, a person may be overweight, with lots of excess fats but lack the essential fat reserves. In fact, obese people actually have low fat reserves, which is very ironic.

The loading days also serve to help prepare better for the burning phase. It help reduce hunger and cravings during the 1st week in the diet. Food addictions and cravings are less intense during the transition period when you will start eating 500 calories per day only.

Those who jump right into the 500 calorie-per-day without loading prove to experience more intense cravings. This eventually get in the way of finishing the 21 to 42 days burning phase. In fact, those who skipped the loading days tend to have more intense cravings and greater challenges within the 1st few days of Phase 2. They also tend to have lower weight loss results within the 1st week of Phase 2.

It only takes 2 days of the loading phase. Don't skip it. Savor it. Aside from the high-calorie fatty foods, you also start taking HCG drops.

HCG PLAN OF LOADING PHASE (PHASE 1)

HCG is started on the loading days. The hormone needs to build up in the body before it can take effect. You have to "load up" on it, too. By the 3rd day of taking HCG, the hormone would have reached its full strength. At this point, HCG will be able to help the body release its fat stores. These stores will fuel the body during the burning phase. This is important because food will only provide 500 calories, way smaller than the average amount of calories needed by the body in a day. The point is to get the body to use its energy stores in the fats. As a result, you lose the excess fats and lose weight- the one that matters.

The loading phase is crucial to weight loss. That may seem counter intuitive as you are eating lots of foods that cause you to become fatter. But that's only for 2 days. This practice proves to be at the core of early, dramatic weight loss within week 1 on the HCG diet plan.

PREPARING FOR THE LOADING PHASE

Proper loading is very important. Women should pick a day that is not very close to the start of the menstrual period. Remember the previous discussion on preparation? Choose at least 10 days before the start of the next menstrual period.

Next, select the foods you load up on. This is the time you eat your most favorite foods. Most likely, this will be the only time you get the chance to. Grab the opportunity. Take this out of the way by loading up on these so you won't feel too deprived once you need to stick to the diet's approved foods list.

The foods must be dense in calories. It is better to load up on fatty foods, as these are denser in calories than grains and carbs. In fact, it is better to stay low carb and go for higher calorie foods like fats and proteins.

Of course, overeating will cause you to gain some weight. Do not worry. This is normal as you will lose all these in Phase 2. The average gain during the loading phase is 1 to 3 pounds. This will be lost generally after Day 1 in the burning phase.

BENEFITS OF THE LOADING PHASE

This phase is preparatory to transitioning from a carb-heavy, processed-loaded diet most of us eat on a daily basis. The body is helped in shifting into a carb-burning machine into a fat-burning efficient system.

Other benefits include:

- Reduces challenges during the entire diet cycle

- Prepares the mind and body for the 500-calorie-a-day burning phase

- Prepares the mind and body for the food restrictions of the next phase

- Helps turn on fat-burning switch

- Reduces hunger during the initial days in the burning phase

- Reduces food addictions and cravings in burning phase

- Reduces frequency and severity of headaches during initial period of burning phase

Improper loading can cause headaches. This is because the body has long been dependent on rapidly digested and absorbed carbs for energy. Fats and proteins are also great energy sources but take a longer time to be digested and absorbed. This delay can cause the tissues to go on low fuel while waiting for energy from fats and proteins.

LOADING PHASE (PHASE 1) MEAL PLAN

This is the fun part of the diet plan. Eat fatty, calorie-rich foods. Eat to capacity. Eat to your heart's content. BUT.... do not eat until you get sick. Just eat until you are full. Do not stuff yourself to the point of sickness.

Take advantage of the loading phase. This is the only phase when you can overeat. Eat the things you love, even the most fattening ones. Pizza, fatty cuts of meat, pasta, rich desserts- eat up.

Why?

The point of the loading phase is to restore any fat reserves missing in the body at this point. The essential fat reserves are the fats that the body needs for protection and for its many homeostatic functions. You see, a person may be overweight, with lots of excess fats but lack the essential fat reserves. In fact, obese people actually have low fat reserves, which is very ironic.

The loading days also serve to help prepare better for the burning phase. It help reduce hunger and cravings during the 1st week in the diet. Food addictions and cravings are less intense during the transition period when you will start eating 500 calories per day only.

Those who jump right into the 500 calorie-per-day without loading prove to experience more intense cravings. This eventually get in the way of finishing the 21 to 42 days burning phase. In fact, those who skipped the loading days tend to have more intense cravings and greater challenges within the 1st few days of Phase 2. They also tend to have lower weight loss results within the 1st week of Phase 2.

It only takes 2 days of the loading phase. Don't skip it. Savor it. Aside from the high-calorie fatty foods, you also start taking HCG drops.

HCG PLAN OF LOADING PHASE (PHASE 1)

HCG is started on the loading days. The hormone needs to build up in the body before it can take effect. You have to "load up" on it, too. By the 3rd day of taking HCG, the hormone would have reached its full strength. At this point, HCG will be able to help the body release its fat stores. These stores will fuel the body during the burning phase. This is important because food will only provide 500 calories, way smaller than the average amount of calories needed by the body in a day. The point is to get the body to use its energy stores in the fats. As a result, you lose the excess fats and lose weight- the one that matters.

The loading phase is crucial to weight loss. That may seem counter intuitive as you are eating lots of foods that cause you to become fatter. But that's only for 2 days. This practice proves to be at the core of early, dramatic weight loss within week 1 on the HCG diet plan.

TIPS FOR LOADING

To help ease the transition, properly load on fats, calories and HCG. A few quick tips can also help:

1. Hydrate. This is very important to keep the headaches and cravings to a minimum. Lots of water also helps flush out additives, food preservatives, free radicals and other toxins from the body. All these can get in the way of creating an efficient fat-burning body.

2. Use high potency, high quality HCG from start to end. Order enough to last from beginning of loading to end of Phase 2.

3. Choose foods with lots of omega-3 fatty acids. These are the foods highly recommended to load up on. Examples are salmon, eggs and nuts such as macadamia.

4. Foods rich in omega-6 fatty acids are may also be added.

WHAT TO EAT

The meal plan is simple in the loading days. It has to be fatty and high in calories. Avoid sugar. There are no strict meal or food lists or any calorie restrictions. The original diet plan by Dr. Simeons was not very specific about food lists during this phase.

Recommended foods to eat, for those who have to idea where to start, are:

- Bread spread with a thick layer of jam and butter
- Fried meats (particularly pork)
- Bacon
- Eggs
- Mayonnaise
- Pastries with whipped cream sugar
- Milk chocolate
- Peanut butter
- Cashews
- Ice cream
- Cheeseburger
- Cheesecake
- Cheese
- Salmon
- Butter
- Steak
- Chicken thighs

Note

Aside from the diet, you should also consider exercise. Continue any exercise you are currently doing. If you aren't exercising at this point, start. Exercise helps in maintaining muscle mass. If you use it, you won't lose it.

Recommended exercise is something low intensity, light impact routine. You can increase it later on. Start with at least 20 minutes of exercise each day. Examples of exercises you can start with are light resistance training, Pilates, swimming, stretching, yoga and brisk walking.

CHAPTER 6: HCG DIET FOR QUICK WEIGHT LOSS

Again, HCG is not the direct and the only aspect that drives weight loss. It is more about the calorie restriction. HCG is a necessary addition because it keeps the body from going into starvation mode that can be triggered by the extreme calorie restriction. Without HCG, the metabolic rate slows down, fat storage rate rises and fat burning almost stops. HCG keeps the metabolism going normally and prevents muscle tissues from getting broken down.

Let's take a closer look at exactly how HCG helps for quick weight loss.

WHAT HAPPENS TO THE BODY DURING RAPID WEIGHT LOSS

Losing weight fast with severe calorie restrictions are usually due to loss of both fat and muscle tissues. Losing muscle mass reflects a huge decrease in scale readings because muscles are heavy. The scale reading may seem great but not for the body.

Muscles play very important roles in metabolism. If muscle mass drops, the body becomes alerted. Muscles must be preserved, especially the proteins and other nutrients stored in it. The body is designed to view drops in muscle mass as a result of extreme starvation.

Theoretically, the body will only metabolize muscles if it has gone too long without adequate calorie intake. It is sort of a last resort to supply the body with its needed nutrients. The body will do what it can to prevent muscle metabolism.

Hence, the body will slow down its metabolic rates. This will reduce the energy spending and energy requirements. It's like shutting off a few appliances to conserve energy consumption in the house.

Calories that are not used by the slowed functioning of the various systems are stored as fats. The body becomes more adamant in salvaging any energy and storing it as fats. This results in increased fat storage. Consequently, the body becomes more resolute in keeping all stored fats. It becomes more determined to limit fat burning.

HCG prevents all these from happening.

Human chorionic gonadotropin is an analogue of many of the body's hormone precursors. It can stimulate various organs in the body to initiate hormonal activities. This includes the thyroid and the adrenal glands. It also influences a woman's ovaries and a man's testes. All other tissues that respond to hormones are affected as well.

HCG helps drive weight loss through several means. It stimulates increased production of progesterone and estrogen, as well as testosterone. All of these 3 hormones are present in males and females, in varying levels. Testosterone is much higher in males than in females. Progesterone and estrogen are much higher in females than in males. All are influenced by HCG. The influence on testosterone plays a major role in the results from HCG treatment.

Testosterone is an important hormone for the muscles. It helps with muscle building. When limiting calorie intake, having small amounts of testosterone helps to preserve the muscle mass. It counteracts the catabolic activity when the body enters a starvation state.

This HCG effect on the levels of testosterone is critical in the diet plan. This plays a central role in body reshaping during the burning phase. This is what makes a huge difference between HCG diet and all other diets. Other diets cause weight loss from both fat and muscle loss. HCG only promotes fat loss, preserving muscle mass. HCG promotes body reshaping, creating leaner muscles instead of muscle shrinking while losing all the unwanted fats. `

HCG PHASE 2- THE BURNING PHASE

Rapid weight loss happens during the diet's Phase 2. This is the crucial stage of the diet. You will be going for 3 to 6 weeks of severe calorie restriction. You will be limited to 500 calories a day only, nothing more. Before you dive into this stage, you must consider your health. Check with the doctor if it is safe for you to be on such very low calorie intake.

Certain conditions may need medical consultation and some allowances. For example, diabetics may need complimentary plans to meet certain needs. A 500-calorie intake unsupervised may predispose them to dangerous hypoglycemia.

Food allergies are also important considerations. If you are allergic to certain foods on Phase 2 list of approved foods, you cannot make any substitutions- unless the substitute is also on the list. The same goes for any items that you do not want to eat based on dietary preferences, health reasons and others.

Getting 500 calories a day can be tough if you eat 3 full meals plus snacks. To reduce the frequency of calorie counting and meal prepping, limit meals to 2 a day.

In creating a meal plan, you have many options. The main thing to remember is never to eat two items from the same category. For example, you are limited to 2 servings of fruit per day. Never take both servings in a meal. For instance, never eat an orange and an apple in the same meal.

TIPS FOR THE BURNING PHASE

Your body will be burning a lot of your excess stored fats during this phase. You can maximize the process with these few tips:

- Hydrate. Aim to drink at least 68 ounces a day. If you weigh more than 136 pounds, get your weight and divide it in half. Take that number and match it in ounces of water. For example, you weigh 200 pounds. Divide it by half, which will be 100. Aim to drink at least 100 ounces of water each day.

- You can drink coffee but limit it to 1-2 cups per day only.

- You can drink tea but check the ingredients first. It should not have any sugar in it. Anything on the packet that ends in -ose means a sugar ingredient. Avoid these kinds of tea.

- London broil and shrimps are allowed during this phase. However, limit it to once a week only. These should be occasional. Never eat both together on the same day.

- Proteins in meals should be mostly from fish and chicken. Avoid tuna.

- Never eat tomatoes and asparagus on the same day. Also, limit consumption of these two. Limit to every 3 to 4 days only.

- Strawberries must be limited to twice a week. Eating too many may cause weight loss to stall.

- Brisk walking and similar activities are good 3 to 4 days a week, an hour each session.

- Do not eat more than 1 apple in a day.

- Grapefruit helps boost fat burning. Eat ½ of a fruit, whether small or large, at a time.

- Rotate foods daily, from proteins, to fruits and vegetables.

- Avoid eating anything within 3 hours of bedtime.

- Avoid OTC medications. Aspirin may be taken when needed.

- Use gloves when preparing food or when using products that may have oils in them.

Be mindful of the last 3 days of the burning phase. Stop taking HCG at this time. However, continue with the rest of the meal plan until the end of the burning phase.

Never skip HCG doses at any time during the burning phase.

Never forget to hydrate adequately. Drink water regularly.

CHAPTER 7:
MAINTENANCE PHASE

After the burning phase comes the maintenance phase. This will last 3 weeks after the burning phase. The goal of this phase is to help the body transition to eating other foods. This phase involves expanding the very limited foods list of Phase 2.

During the maintenance phase, avoid sugars and starches. The body needs to stabilize after the intense calorie restriction of the burning phase. The starches and sugars are gradually introduced as the maintenance phase ends.

Weight is still taken every morning. If the scale readings reflect weight gain greater than 2 pounds, skip a meal for the day. This will help the body to gain better control over weight and appetite.

Rules for the maintenance phase according to Dr. Simeons' original diet plan are:

- Weigh every day, best in the morning. Empty the bladder first (urinate) before weighing.

- Monitor weight and keep it within 2 pounds of the last injection weight (weight on the last day of HCG injection).

- Eat lots of true proteins every day, at least 100 grams. This will be around 400 grams of actual meat (weight taken while still raw). That is, to get 100 grams real protein, that will be eating 400 grams of beef, weighed just before cooking.

The weight will generally stabilize towards the end of the 3-week period. This means that there will be no large fluctuations in the weight for a few consecutive days.

Remember to avoid starches and sugars. If meals for the day contain zero carbs, you can indulge in fats with relative liberality. That is, you can eat more fats but not to the point of excess, getting sick or too full to move. Alcohol in small quantities may also be added on zero-carb days. You can take 1 glass of wine with one of the day's meals.

Again, indulging must still be with control.

WHEN TO START THE MAINTENANCE PHASE

This phase starts 72 hours after giving the last injection or drops for the burning phase. For example, the last dose was taken at 9AM on Monday. The maintenance phase starts on Thursday, 9AM. It is not after 3 days but exactly after 72 hours.

During the 72-hour period between the last HCG dose and the beginning of Phase 3, follow the 500-calorie-a-day VLCD (very low calorie diet). Some variations of the HCG Diet classify this 72-hour period as an additional phase.

The rules in the maintenance phase must be strictly followed as in the other phases. At this point, the body is in reset. The hypothalamus is functioning in its normal state, without the distractions of too much carb in the diet.

Remember to highlight the weight you took on the morning of your last HCG dose. This will be your baseline weight for the maintenance phase. You should stay within 2 pounds of this weight. If your weight on any day of the maintenance phase reflects an increase of more than 2 pounds of the last HCG dose weight, plan your day's meal to focus more on proteins. Eliminate any carbs and sugars. Any food that might contain any of these must be avoided for the rest of the day. If you must drink water alone instead of coffee and other beverages, do so. Avoid sugars and starches.

GUIDELINES TO THE MAINTENANCE PHASE

Again, maintenance phase is 72 hours after the last dose of HCG. Calorie intake increases to at least 1500. Never continue the 500 calorie-a-day diet once HCG is out of the body.

Remember how HCG plays an important role in diets with severely restricted calorie intake? It keeps the body from going into starvation mode.

If you continue the 500 calories without the HCG, you will slow down metabolism and trigger starvation mode. The result? Losing everything you have worked hard for.

So, back to maintenance phase.

Weight is expected to fluctuate during this phase. Just remember to monitor it and it should not exceed a 2-ppound weight gain.

Absolutely no starch and sugar.

Eat enough. This is no longer a calorie-restricted diet phase. You do not have to eat as if you need to keep calories low. Eat as you normally would when not on a weight loss diet. Just remember to eat within the approved list and no sugar and starch.

If you need to increase your calories, add more dairy products and healthy fats.

Remember to hydrate properly and get enough sleep.

CHAPTER 8:
HCG DIET DAILY MEAL PLAN

The daily meal plan of this diet differs among the phases. It is important to follow the meal plans because it is the carefully planned meals that bring about the rapid weight loss. In addition, you have to take the HCG doses as instructed to keep the body from reacting to the calorie restrictions. Again, diet drives the weight loss, HCG keeps the body from fighting the rapid weight loss and losing muscle mass.

PHASE 1 LOADING DAYS

Sample Meal Plan

Breakfast (any of the following)

- 2 sausage links

- 2 bacon slices

- Ham and cheese omelet (using 2 whole eggs, heavy cream, cheese, ham and butter)

- Toasted bagel with cream cheese

These simple breakfast choices can give the body around 100 grams of fat.

Lunch *(any of the following)*

- Large servings of fatty meats such as pork ribs, pork chops, rib-eye steak or regular ground beef, roasted with lots of oil or sautéed in butter

- Fish or lean cuts of poultry fried or cooked then served with cream- or butter-based sauce or simply with a few pats of seasoned or herbed butter

- Pair meats with thick buttered rolls, vegetables cooked in oil or butter, baked potato with butter and sour cream

Dinner *(any of the following)*

- Pasta, with regular noodles and heavy Alfredo sauce, a side of buttered French bread with shredded cheese and salad topped with full-fat dressing

- Salads with cream-based or oil-based dressing, topped with crunchy bacon bits

- Diced avocados and hard-boiled eggs

- Cheesecake for dessert

Snacks *(any of the following)*

Snacks during the loading phase are highly recommended. Get at least 2-3 snacks in between meals.

- Doughnuts with whipped cream

- Milkshakes, fast-food or homemade

- Full fat ice cream

- Pastries

- Crackers with peanut butter spread

- Candies

- Chocolate bars

- French fries with melted cheese and bacon bits

- Macadamia nuts or other nuts

HCG Diet Loading Days Foods List

- Avocados

- Olives

- Avocado oil

- Olive oils

- Salmon

- Mackerel

- Tuna

- Herring

- Sardines

- Lake trout

- Almonds

- Macadamia nuts

- Walnuts

- Hazelnuts

- Brazil nuts

- Peanuts

- Natural or organic peanut butter

- Flax seed oil

- Pumpkin seeds

- Flax seeds

- Sunflower seeds

- Heavy cream

- Whole eggs

- Hurricane mayo

- Cheese

- Cottage cheese

PHASE 2 BURNING PHASE

Sample Meal Plan

A typical daily meals in the burning phase consists of the following menu:

Breakfast (any of the following)

(Tea or coffee with one serving of fruit)

- Coffee mixed with 1 tablespoon 2% milk and a touch of Stevia plus 1 medium orange

- 1 liter water and 1 apple

Lunch *(any of the following)*

(100 grams of one of the approved proteins, 1 starch, 1 vegetable, and 1 fruit)

- 100 grams lean beef patty with 1 tomato (sliced) and 1 tablespoon mustard

- 1 serving beef stew and ½ of a medium-sized apple

- 00 grams baked orange roughy with 2 full glasses of water

Dinner *(any of the following)*

(100 grams of any one approved protein, 1 vegetable, 1 fruit and 1 starch)

- 1 serving Chesapeake crab soup

- 100 grams tilapia cooked with lemon juice, 2 melba snacks and 6 steamed asparagus spears plus ½ apple

- 100 grams canned tuna served with lettuce leaves and fresh herb dressing

- 100 grams boiled shrimp with crispy onion rings, 1 Melba toast and 1 handful of blueberries

At times, it may surprise you that you do not feel hungry even with the severe calorie restriction. This is OK. You may skip the starch, vegetable or fruit from your meals.

However, never skip the protein part. This is very important because your body is being trained to use fats and proteins as sources of energy. The fat source will be from the fat stores your body is burning,. The protein source will be from your meals.

Again, never skip the protein. You can skip everything else if you feel you are not up to it.

Desserts may be added to meals. This is usually taken during dinnertime.

- Strawberries and cream

- Apple compote with melba toast

Snacks may also be allowed. Just check that you make room for it and not go beyond 500 calories for the day.

Snacks *(any of the following)*

- 2 melba toasts

- Handful of berries

- 1 apple

HCG Diet Burning Phase Foods List

Proteins

During this phase, proteins should not exceed 200 grams daily. Limit proteins to not more than 100 mg proteins in one meal. Remove all visible fat from the protein source. Bones should be removed before cooking the meat.

Approved protein sources during Phase 2 are:

- Chicken

- 3 Egg Whites

- Extra Lean Beef

- White Fish

- Scallops

- Crab

- Lobster

- Shrimp

- Buffalo

Vegetables

Phase 2 puts importance on vegetables but should still be in controlled quantities. Only 2 meals in a day should include 1 cup of vegetables. That will be a total of 2 cups of vegetables per day. Remember, 1 cup per meal, 2 meals in a day. Never take more than 1 cup of vegetables in one meal and never more than 2 cups in a day.

Approved vegetables are:

- Salad Greens

- Celery

- Fennel

- Red Radishes

- Cucumbers

- Cauliflower

- Broccoli

- Onions

- Shallots

- Tomatoes

- Spinach

- Beet Greens

- Cabbage

- Mixed Greens

- Chard

- Asparagus

Fruits

These are healthy but most contain large amounts of sugar. Phase 2 allows fruits but in limited amounts. This phase recommends eating fruits daily but should not exceed 2 servings per day.

Allowed fruits in Phase 2 are:

- Grapefruit

- Apples

- Oranges

- Lemons

- Raspberries

- Blueberries

- Strawberries

Miscellaneous Items

A few additional items are allowed in the Phase 2. These items can be added to food to enhance flavors.

Allowed miscellaneous items in Phase 2 are:

- Salt, pepper, or any other natural spices

- Apple Cider Vinegar

- Mustard powder

- Braggs Amino Acids

- Coffee

- Herbal Tea

- Stevia

Never use dressings, butter or oil on anything. Seasoning mixes must be avoided as well. These contain too much salt and sugar.

PHASE 3 MAINTENANCE PHASE

Sample Menu Plan

Breakfast

- Mixed berries with stevia and Greek yogurt and 2 eggs

- Vegetable omelette made with sautéed bell peppers, tomatoes, mushrooms and onions, with 2 eggs topped with 2 tablespoons shredded cheese

- Meaty omelette with turkey bacon, bell peppers, mushrooms, onions and Parmesan cheese

Lunch

- Burger patty with pickles, tomato, lettuce and mustard, served with a side salad

- Grilled salmon topped with creamed spinach

- Tuna salad lettuce wrap

Dinner

- Lettuce taco- normal taco but replace tortilla with large lettuce leaves

- Chuck roast steak kabobs with pearl onions and button mushrooms

- Baked chicken breast with side salad and steamed green beans

Snacks

- Apple slices with peanut butter

- Mixed nuts

- Pear

- 2 kiwi

HCG Maintenance Phase Allowed Foods List

Proteins

All fishes are allowed such as:

- Salmon

- Tuna

- Sardines

- Herring

- Sole

- Trout

- Flounder

All poultry sources are allowed such as:

- Chicken

- Cornish hen

- Turkey

- Goose

- Duck

- Quail

- Pheasant

All shellfish are allowed such as:

- Shrimp

- Scallops

- Clams

- Oysters*

- Mussels*

- Crab Meat

- Squid

* Mussels and oysters contain higher carbs, so servings should be limited to around 4 ounces per day.

All meat sources are allowed such as:

- Lean beef

- Pork

- Lamb

- Ham*

- Bacon*

- Venison

- Lean bison

- Veal

*Some bacon, ham and processed meat is cured using sugar. This adds to the carbohydrate count. Some of these may still be safe to include in Phase 3. Look at the grams sugar per serving. Choose those with zero grams sugar. Avoid meats and cold cuts with added nitrates.

Vegetables

(Salad Vegetables)

- Romaine lettuce

- Iceberg lettuce

- Alfalfa sprouts

- Parsley

- Chives

- Arugula

- Celery

- Bok choy

- Chicory greens

- Fennel

- Endive

- Mushrooms

- Escarole

- Radicchio

- Cucumber

- Radishes

- Peppers

(Non-salad vegetables)

- Spinach

- Kale

- Collard Greens

- Tomato

- Swiss Chard

- Leeks

- Cabbage

- Asparagus
- Artichokes
- Brussels Sprouts
- Artichoke Hearts
- Olives (black & green)
- Cauliflower
- Broccoli
- Peas
- Eggplant
- Okra
- Rhubarb
- Onion
- Bamboo Shoots
- Spaghetti squash
- Summer Squash
- Pumpkin
- Water Chestnuts
- Turnips
- Zucchini
- Hearts of Palm
- Sauerkraut

*Non-salad vegetables contain slightly more carbs than salad vegetables. However, these are still great additions to meals as these provide important nutrients. These also add variety to make daily meals more flavorful.

Fruits

- Fresh blueberries

- Fresh strawberries

- Fresh raspberries

- Honeydew or cantaloupe

Fats

- Butter, real not margarine or imitation butter

- Mayonnaise, no added sugar or make your own

- Avocado Oil

- Olive Oil

- Coconut Oil

Oils

- Coconut oil

- Flax seed oil

- Grape seed oil

- Walnut oil

- Sesame oil

- Canola oil

- Sunflower oil

- Safflower Oil

Dairy

- Heavy cream

- Cow, goat, and sheep cheese

- Cottage cheese

- Mozzarella cheese

- Blue cheeses

- Ricotta cheese

- Cream cheese

- Cheddar

- Feta

- Parmesan

- Mozzarella

- Gouda

- Swiss

CHAPTER 9: HCG RECIPES

MAIN DISHES

Roasted Onions and Steak

Ingredients

- 100 grams flank steak

- Seasoning of choice, must be within the diet's allowed list

- 1 small onion, sliced

Directions

1. Preheat the oven to broil temperature.

2. Season the steak.

3. Brown the steak on both sides in a hot skillet.

4. Place on a baking sheet.

5. Put the steak in the preheated oven. Broil to desired doneness.

6. In the same skillet, add a splash of water and the onion slices.

7. Sauté until translucent.

8. Place cooked steak on a plate. Top with sautéed onions.

Apple Chicken Wraps

Ingredients

- 100 grams diced chicken

- dash of pepper, smoked paprika, and salt

- 1 small apple diced

- 2 tablespoons of lemon juice

- 1/8 teaspoon cardamom

- 1/8 teaspoon cinnamon

- Sprinkle of stevia

Directions

1. Put chicken into a hot skillet.

2. Add a dash each of salt, pepper and smoked paprika. Sauté until chicken is cooked through. Set aside on a serving plate.

3. Put diced apples in a mixing bowl.

4. Add lemon juice, cardamom and cinnamon. Toss.

5. Add to the plate, beside the diced chicken. Sprinkle with a small amount of stevia.

6. Serve.

Whitefish Taco

Ingredients

- 100 grams of whitefish
- Juice squeezed from ½ lemon
- 1 clove crushed garlic
- ½ teaspoon chili powder
- ¼ teaspoon ground cumin
- Dash of salt
- Cracked black pepper to taste

Directions

1. Heat oven to 350 degrees Fahrenheit.
2. Pour lemon juice over the fish.
3. Mix all spices in a small bowl. Sprinkle over he fish.
4. Turn the fish to coat all sides with spice mix.
5. Put fish on a baking tray. Bake until fish easily flakes.
6. Once done, flake the fish and serve over a bed of iceberg lettuce leaves.

SOUPS AND SALADS

Asparagus Soup

Ingredients

- 4-5 asparagus stems

- 2 tablespoons fresh lemon juice

- 2 tablespoons white onion

- 1 cup chicken broth

- ½ teaspoon dill

- ½ teaspoon onion powder

- Salt & pepper, adjusted to liking

Procedure

1. Steam asparagus stems until tender. Cool slightly then puree in a blender with the onion.

2. Pour asparagus-onion puree into a pot. Add the rest of the ingredients.

3. Heat soup over medium flame until warmed all throughout. Serve.

Beef Stew

(Serve with 1 piece of Melba toast, to dip into the soup)

Ingredients

- 100 g steak, sliced into chunks
- 1 ½ cups beef broth
- 2 tablespoons diced onion
- 1 bay leaf
- 1 ¼ cup chopped celery
- 2 minced garlic cloves
- ¼ teaspoon rosemary
- ¼ teaspoon garlic powder
- Salt & pepper, adjusted to liking

Procedure

1. Season steak chunks with pepper, garlic powder and salt. Mix and out in a small pot.

2. Add minced garlic and onions. Set pot over medium-high flame and lightly sauté steak until browned.

3. Add the rest of the ingredients. Allow to simmer on low flame for 45 minutes.

4. Add water and more pepper and salt as desired.

5. Discard bay leaf. Serve hot.

Cabbage & Beef Soup

Ingredients

- 100 g lean steak, sliced small

- 1 ½ cups beef broth

- 1 tablespoon chopped green onion

- 2 tablespoons chopped onion

- ½ teaspoon garlic powder

- ¼ teaspoon dried basil

- ½ teaspoon ground ginger

- 1 cup shredded cabbage

- Salt & pepper, added to liking

Procedure

1. Mix steak with garlic powder, ginger, pepper and salt.

2. Sauté the seasoned steak in 2 tablespoons of the beef broth until steak is lightly browned.

3. Add shredded cabbage and sauté for about 1 minute.

4. Add the remaining ingredients and simmer soup for 30 to 45 minutes.

5. Serve hot.

Chesapeake Crab Soup

Ingredients

- 100 g cooked crab
- 1 ½ cups vegetable broth
- 1 ½ tomatoes, diccd
- 1 minced garlic clove
- 2 tablespoons chopped onion
- 1-2 teaspoons Old Bay Seasoning
- Pepper & salt, adjusted to liking

Procedure

1. Put all ingredients in a pot. Set over medium high flame and bring to a boil.
2. Reduce flame to a simmer and cook for 15 minutes.
3. Serve hot.

Chili

Ingredients

- 1 pound lean ground beef
- 1 ½ cups water
- 3 cups chopped tomatoes
- ½ cup chopped onion

- ½ teaspoon oregano

- 4 minced garlic cloves

- 1 teaspoon onion powder

- 1 teaspoon garlic powder

- 1 teaspoon chili powder

- Cayenne pepper, adjusted to liking

- Salt & pepper, adjusted to liking

Procedure

1. Sauté beef until browned. Add minced garlic and chopped onions. Sauté until fragrant.

2. Add tomatoes, spices and water. Allow soup to simmer for 20-30 minutes.

3. Serve hot topped with some chopped green onions.

Cucumber Vinegar Salad

Ingredients

- 1 cucumber, cubed

- ¼ cup white vinegar

- ¼ teaspoon onion salt

- Fresh ground pepper

- 2 teaspoons chopped fresh parsley

- 2 teaspoons chopped green onion

- Stevia, add to liking

Procedure

1. Place all ingredients in a mixing bowl. Toss to coat.

2. Serve.

Cucumber Grapefruit Salad

Ingredients

- 1 cucumber, cubed

- 1 ruby red grapefruit, sliced in half

- 1 tablespoon diced small purple onion

- 1 tablespoon chopped green onion

- Handful of fresh cilantro, finely chopped

- Salt & pepper, added to liking

Ruby Red Dressing

- Remaining grapefruit juice from halves

- 2 tablespoons apple cider vinegar

- ½ teaspoon fresh ginger

- Salt & pepper, added to liking

- Orange Stevia, added to liking

Procedure

1. Scoop out grapefruit sections. Put in a mixing bowl.

2. Squeeze out juice from the remaining halves. Out juice in a separate small mixing bowl.

3. Add onions into the grapefruit sections. Mix in pepper, cilantro, cucumber and salt. mix.

4. Combine ingredients for Ruby Red dressing. Pour over salad.

5. Toss then serve.

SIDES

Sliced Tomato Roast

Ingredients

- 1 tomato, sliced into rounds
- garlic salt, to season
- 1 sprig rosemary, coarsely chopped
- 1 crushed garlic clove

Directions

1. Preheat the oven to 200 degrees Fahrenheit.
2. Line a baking tray with parchment paper.
3. Arrange the tomato slices in a single layer on the prepared baking tray.
4. Sprinkle the slices with rosemary and garlic salt.
5. Place the crushed garlic clove in between the tomato slices.
6. Roast in the oven for an hour.

Dill Cucumber Salad

Ingredients

- 1 medium cucumber sliced then quartered
- 1 teaspoon dill

- 1 tablespoon vinegar

- Stevia to taste

- Black pepper

Directions

1. Put cucumbers in a serving bowl.

2. Mix dill and vinegar in a separate small bowl.

3. Season with stevia and black pepper. Stir well and pour over cucumbers.

4. Stir a little just to mix evenly.

5. Serve.

Oven-Roasted Asparagus

Ingredients

- 1 bunch of asparagus

- 1 tablespoon lemon juice

- 3 tablespoons water

- 1 teaspoon salt

- 1 minced garlic clove

- black pepper to taste

Directions

1. Heat the oven to 425 degrees Fahrenheit.

2. Mix water and lemon juice.

3. Put asparagus in a mixing bowl. Pour over the water-lemon juice mixture. Toss to coat evenly.

4. Spread the asparagus in a single layer on a baking tray.

5. Sprinkle salt and minced garlic. Season to taste with cracked black pepper.

6. Bake until done to preferred tenderness. Serve immediately.

BEVERAGES

Strawberry Slushy

Ingredients

- 5 fresh strawberries

- 1 cup crushed ice

- Stevia to taste

- 1 teaspoon vanilla extract

Directions

1. Use a blender to blend strawberries, vanilla and ice until a slushy appearance is formed.

2. Sweeten to taste with stevia. Blend just to mix and pour into a glass.

Blended Coffee

Ingredients

- 2 cups ice

- 1 cup strong coffee

- Stevia to taste

Directions

1. Place ice and strong coffee in a blender. Blend well.

2. Sweeten to taste with stevia.

3. Pour into a glass and enjoy.

4. Add flavors as preferred, such as peppermint, chocolate, cinnamon and the likes.

Grapefruit Spritzer

Ingredients

- 8 oz. sparking mineral water

- Juice from 1 grapefruit

- Crushed ice

- Orange stevia drops, according to taste

Directions

1. Pour grapefruit juice in a small bowl. Add orange stevia according to preferred sweetness. Stir.

2. Pour mixture into sparkling mineral water and stir gently.

3. Pour mixture over a glass filled with crushed ice.

DESSERTS

Chocolate Cheesecake

Ingredients

- 1 tablespoon cocoa powder

- 100 g no-fat or low-fat cottage cheese

- Liquid stevia, adjusted to taste

- Splash of vanilla extract

Directions

1. Put all ingredients in a blender or food processor to puree until smooth. Adjust stevia to taste.

2. Pour into a ramekin. Garnish with any of the allowed fruits.

Strawberries with Cream

Ingredients

- Fresh strawberries, sliced

- 2-4 drops vanilla creme Stevia

- 1 tablespoon milk

- 1 packet powdered Stevia

Procedure

1. Mix all the ingredients.

2. Serve chilled.

CHAPTER 10: COMMON FAQS

Can loading days be 3 instead of 2?

Yes. In fact, the original diet plan by Dr. Simeons sometimes used 7 days as loading days. However, the 7-day loading period is only for people who have low fat intake for a very long time.

For most other people, 2 to 3 days of loading is OK. Best results were observed among those who kept loading days to 2 only.

A 3rd day may be added if you feel one of the loading days haven't been successful. Should you add a 3rd day to the loading phase, take HCG on the 3rd as well.

What to do if I lose some weight during the loading phase?

This usually means that you are not eating enough. If this happens, add a 3rd day to your loading phase. Choose foods that are high in fat, not on carbs.

If you continue to lose weight on loading days despite high fat, calorie dense foods and adding a 3rd loading day, that's fine. Time to proceed to the next phase, the burning phase or Phase 2.

Normally, weight gain happens in the loading phase. This is lost at the end of the 1st day of the burning phase. This is if the loading was done properly.

If loading was correct and weight is lost, do not fret. Move on to the next phase and be content you had a head start.

What is the acceptable weight gain during loading?

There are no hard rules on how much you can gain while loading. This is not the period to be overly concerned about weight. Gain as much weight during the loading days. Again, these will all come off on the next phase.

On the average, around 1 to 3 pounds might be gained in Phase 1.

How fast can I lose the loading weight?

The rates are different. Some people can lose more during the first day on Phase 2 while some may take 2 to 3 days. Generally, weight loss during the initial week of phase 2 is about 8-12 pounds. This includes the weight gained during the loading phase.

Some dieters get to lose all the load weight gain and some more right at the end of the 1st day of the burning phase. Some may only lose the load weight. Most of the weight loss is from water weight, not so much as fat weight. However, at this point, fat is starting to be burned for energy so there is still some notable weight loss from fats.

CHAPTER 11:
THE INJECTION PHOBIA

The original HCG diet by Dr. Simeons called for HCG injections. This mode of administering HCG has many benefits. One of the most important benefit is that 100% of the HCG dose injected gets absorbed by the body. With drops, a significant percentage gets deactivated and eventually excreted by the body. Only a few gets to be absorbed and used by the tissues.

If you check the dosage recommendations on HCG preparations, the oral drops come with much higher dosages than injected forms. This is to compensate for the percentage of HCG that becomes inactive and excreted.

Injections are given daily. The HCG is usually already contained in predetermined doses inside small insulin syringes. Just take 1 syringe and inject. Some injectable forms may need mixing right at the time of injection. Carefully read the manufacturer's instructions.

Generally, HCG will come with its own mixing solution. Use this and never substitute anything for it. Withdraw the appropriate amount of mixing solution then inject it into the vial containing the HCG. The amount is usually 5ml mixing solution to the HCG vial. Roll the HCG vial between the palms or swirl it gently to mix the solution. Never shake the vial. This will create bubbles and bubbles in injections are never a good thing. Once mixed well, withdraw 0.2 ml (20 mark on the insulin syringe) of the HCG mixture.

Mix one vial at a time. A vial usually contains multiple doses. Finish a vial first before mixing another one. If not, the potency of the other vials might be affected if it sits too long unused.

If unsure, consult a doctor and seek proper guidance on how to mix and inject HCG.

The most accessible and easiest spot to inject HCG is the abdominal area. Place an ice bag over the area before injecting. This will help numb the area a little and reduce the pain.

Pinch a small area of the stomach. Wipe it with alcohol. Aim the needle at the center of this area. The needle should be injected perpendicular to the surface of the skin. Insert the needle in one swift careful motion. Inject the HCG into the tissue.

Remove the needle and release the stomach area from your pinch. Press down on the injected area for a few seconds.

WHAT ABOUT INJECTION PHOBIA?

Some people are uneasy around needles. Some are plainly terrified of it. For these people, oral drops may be taken instead.

However, remember that the diet is originally designed for HCG injections. The results were obtained from this type of HCG administration.

Oral drops may still work, as seen in many dieters who chose this method. However, the potency and the success rate will not be as great as when using injections.

ANY SIDE EFFECTS?

As with other stuff you give your body, there might be a few side effects. Some people experience these, some don't. severity and duration also vary. Some side effects are only during the initial period.

A few of the noted side effects include:

- Pain over the pelvic and stomach area

- Acne

- Vomiting

- Diarrhea

- Minor bloating

- Pain over the ovaries

- Irregularities in monthly periods

- Breast tenderness

- Headaches

- Irritability

- Moments of shortness of breath

- Gynecomastia in men (enlargement of breasts)

- Excessive sweating in the hands and legs

Should any of these increase in severity, consult a doctor. If taking injections, minor swelling, pain and irritation in the injected area is normal as a result of the invasive procedure. However, if these increase in severity or does not go away after a few minutes, consult a doctor.

CONCLUSION

Thank you for reading this book.

I hope you have gained a better understanding of what HCG is and what the HCG diet can do for you.

Should you decide to follow the diet protocol, take note of all the guidelines, rules, tips and precautions. It is always a good thing to consult a doctor prior to the diet, during and after the diet. Always be aware of how your body reacts. If you do not feel good, do not hesitate to consult a doctor.

Again, thank you for downloading this book.

I hope you find this book enlightening and helpful in your quest for safe and effective weight loss.

Success comes from strict adherence to the protocol. Adjustments may be enforced as long as it is done with proper consideration of all factors involved and with the help of a doctor.

Thank you and good luck!

82957765R00047

Made in the USA
San Bernardino, CA
19 July 2018